Senior's Tai Chi Workout

Improve Balance, Strength, and Flexibility

Master Domingo Colon

The Tai Chi School of Westchester, est. 1978

www.taichischool.com

Order this book online at www.trafford.com
or email orders@trafford.com

Most Trafford titles are also available at major online book retailers.

Print information available on the last page.

ISBN: 978-1-4120-7764-4 (sc)
ISBN: 978-1-4122-0256-5 (e)

Library of Congress Control Number: 2009940190

Trafford rev. 03/20/2017

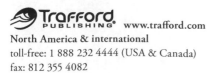

www.trafford.com

North America & international
toll-free: 1 888 232 4444 (USA & Canada)
fax: 812 355 4082

Disclaimer

Neither the author nor the publisher assumes any responsibility for the use or misuse of the information contained in this book.

Even though the practice of Tai Chi, when performed as instructed and described herein, is extremely safe, it is suggested that you consult your doctor or other health professional to determine if the exercises in this book are appropriate for you at this time.

Since your health professional may not be familiar with these Tai Chi exercises, it would be helpful in their evaluation if you let them see this book. Any inquiries from your health professional may be directed to Master Domingo Colon at **sifu@taichischool.com** and will be answered promptly.

Dedication

Dedicated to all seniors, Tai Chi students and non-students, who continually strive to maximize what they are capable of and actively work to improve and maintain a healthy lifestyle of body and mind, as nature intended.

They truly believe and live the saying, **"Use it or lose it!"**

Acknowledgements

Profound thanks to all who have assisted me in the past and inspired me to explore Tai Chi and other health systems to effectively help others improve their health in body and mind.

Special thanks to:

Tai Chi Masters C K Chu, B P Chan, and Wm C C Chen, for sharing their Tai Chi knowledge.

All of my assistant teachers and those individuals that I have had the privilege of promoting to teachers, for constantly challenging me to refine my knowledge and teaching methods.

All of my physical therapy instructors and associates for promoting a balance of eastern and western healing methods.

All who contributed to creating this book:
    Editing, layout, etc. with extra gratitude to:
        Nicola Briggs, cover photography,
        John Horne, all other photography,
        Jay Ballesteros, cover design.

My wonderful seniors who posed for photos:
        Loretta McFarlane
        Hilde Reiter
        Sally Froelich

And all who provided support on so many different levels.

Table of Contents

Forward

Time marks the body. Although this is an inevitable fact of growing older, many people feel that this is a negative statement from which there is no "recovery." However, if we truly consider life to be a cycle, we can have faith in rebounding after a period of inactivity, illness or injury at any age.

Our body naturally desires movement, and we can nurture and heal ourselves every day by giving it what it wants!

One of the most effective ways of turning back the tide, physically and mentally, is to practice Tai Chi.

How would you like to wake up every day without feeling an ounce of stiffness?

Would you like to learn how to move with the grace and flexibility of a cat?

How would you like to walk without any fear of falling?

Most of all, wouldn't it be delightful to simply have more strength and energy to do everything you want to do, to live your life to the fullest degree possible?

We all have the same answers to these questions, but often don't have the method, the concrete know-how, to really help ourselves.

That's where this guide comes in handy -showing you step-by-step the essential movements of Tai Chi so that you can get right to the heart of improving your balance, increasing your bone density and building more muscle in every part of your body.

My teacher and mentor, Master Domingo Colon, has carefully designed every aspect of this course from his 40+ years of experience in Tai Chi and training in physical therapy, specializing in improving mobility in older adults.

From my time as an apprentice with him, I have personally seen how he takes the time needed to address fully each student's challenges, and this detailed approach has been carried over into the *Senior's Tai Chi Workout*. In this book, he has introduced a modern sense of clarity to these ancient, traditional exercises that greatly improves their accessibility to the general public.

The included exercises are like diamonds - handed down to us in the rough through the mists of time, and then cut and polished to a high sheen by each talented interpreter. For without this keen eye, their beauty would be indecipherable.

Master Colon has long believed that an important part of learning and appreciating Tai Chi is to know with the utmost specificity, "How will this exercise help me?" When we understand what the benefits are, we tend to adhere to practice more, which in turn, yields even further benefit. This knowledge really helps to keep the "eyes on the prize," giving you motivation when you need it most.

You will find that the process of learning Tai Chi movement is one of constant renewal and self-discovery. Just when you thought you didn't have the strength or balance to do another "Crane kicks out," you surprise yourself by doing two more.

If you're an "A" type personality who couldn't envision moving slowly, you start to gradually realize that it's much healthier to be like a bicycle with many working gears, not just the ones that let you race at your usual break-neck pace.

Not only does Tai Chi give you greater coordination and flexibility, but also it changes you in another very fundamental way. It improves the circulation of blood, energy, and lymphatic fluids throughout your body, and strengthens your entire immune system, therefore your chances of becoming ill decrease dramatically.

Practicing Tai Chi also wards off depression and brings a deeply calming influence into your life. With each exercise learned, you will have placed in your virtual medicine cabinet one more powerful antidote that you can regularly call upon for preventive and healing purposes.

Glowing health and vitality is certainly within our grasp, and all we have to do is reach out and grab it!

So remember that old adage, "You're only as young as you feel," and encourage your young nature by learning these beautiful movements.

Nicola Briggs
Head Tai Chi Instructor
Tai Chi School of Westchester, est. 1978
September 2005

Preface

I started my own journey into Tai Chi with Master Colon over 10 years ago. As a medical doctor, I was looking for a serious exercise regimen that would logically fit with my knowledge of the principles of health and body mechanics.

After trying other exercises, I came to Tai Chi because of the extensive scientific literature supporting Tai Chi as an exercise that could be done well into my senior years. I was attracted to studying Tai Chi with Master Domingo Colon, because of his years of training as a Physical Therapist, an Adaptive Fitness Specialist, and at the time, 30 + years of Tai Chi experience.

By combining Tai Chi practice along with modern therapeutic principles, Master Colon has created a unique health program accessible to elderly adults, including those with a range of health problems.

Tai Chi movements incorporate balance, flexibility, and toning through slow, graceful actions. Consistent practice of this gentle art has proven to have multiple health benefits, including reduced incidence of cardiovascular diseases such as coronary heart disease and stroke. Tai Chi helps boost the immune system, improve digestion, and decrease depression, all while promoting relaxation. Further studies suggest that the elderly can reduce risk of falls, lower blood pressure and ease Osteo- and Rheumatoid Arthritis symptoms with Tai Chi.

Other significant benefits include increased strength, better balance, and superior coordination, compared to non-Tai Chi practitioners. This minimizes the risk of falling, and enables one to reach into the top cupboard with confidence. Good leg strength makes it easier to get up from a sitting position, and strong lungs mean that one can walk without becoming winded.

Yet as the body ages, vigorous exercise becomes challenging. Tai Chi offers a safe and effective way for even frail elderly adults to improve respiratory health, trunk control, balance, and coordination by incorporating all of the motions that typically become more difficult with aging. This is an ancient way to regain some of the physical functioning that may have been lost due to inactivity.

Even though Tai Chi is one of the safest exercises around, seniors interested in learning should seek out a class specifically designed for them, such as this program. In Master Colon's *Workbook*, students are trained to work within their capabilities as they practice the forms, which involve standing on one leg or walking with a narrow stance, for instance. Students practice recognizing and maintaining stable footing until they develop a firm base and corresponding ability to balance.

I highly recommend this program for all mature adults at all levels of fitness as a superior method to improve and maintain health and physical ability.

Dr. James Horne, DO
Medical Director
Mercy First
New York, New York

December 2005

Introduction and welcome to Tai Chi

You are about to begin an exciting journey to increased **health, strength,** and **peace of mind**.

This book is designed to make it easy for you to benefit from the ancient art of Tai Chi. Therefore; you will find clear and complete instructions in how to perform a fundamental workout that includes all basic aspects of Tai Chi for health. You may perform this workout daily, with no strain, and continue to develop and improve your health.

The principles and concepts of Tai Chi are presented efficiently in a clear and concise manner to avoid overwhelming you with detail and unnecessary Chinese language and terminology. Learning and doing Tai Chi will be an enjoyable experience for you; you will look forward to every practice session with enthusiasm.

By following these simple exercises practiced by millions of Chinese people for over a thousand years, you are joining the countless people seen in the graceful performance of these gentle movements on a daily basis in the parks, plazas and streets of China, and increasingly throughout the world.

Gently and gradually, you will move through the beginning stages of Tai Chi and absorb this wonderful art form easily into your body and mind with a minimum of effort.

Tai Chi is a unique system of health and self-defense developed centuries ago in China. Therefore, this approach to fitness is quite different from any you may have experienced.

Tai Chi is not about memorizing a series of movements, but about becoming aware of your body and mind thereby eliminating bad habits that stand in your way to outstanding health.

In learning Tai Chi, two principal stages that you will experience are the *yin* phase and the *yang* phase. Although understanding *yin* and *yang*, the duality that exists in all of nature, can be a complex theory to absorb, at this time let us say that, as an example of this duality, learning the choreography or the mechanics of Tai Chi represents the *yang* phase. Then, the development of the correct **feeling** or **quality** of these movements represents the *yin* phase.

In order to maximize your benefits, you need to pay attention to both phases; concentrate first on learning the correct technique (*yang*), then focus on developing the proper feeling of the movements (*yin*).

Take your time to experience these movements deeply and understand the underlying principles and you will be able to make Tai Chi an important part of your everyday life. Consistent review and refinement will provide you with all of the benefits that you are looking for and more.

Please remember: Your priority should be how well you perform and feel the movements, within your personal ability, not how many exercises you learn.

The object of Tai Chi is to effect a profound transformation of your body and mind, not merely the rote memorization of a sequence of movements, as is so often the case in other exercise classes.

Concentrate on the few basics given to establish a strong foundation for continued future development. As you do Tai Chi, you will condition your body, becoming stronger, more flexible, better coordinated, improving your breathing and gaining many other benefits. All this takes time. Please be patient with yourself and enjoy the process.

Focus on slow, gentle, and relaxed movements-each flowing into the next without strain. Breathe normally and in a relaxed manner until you can comfortably perform the precise breathing method associated with each exercise.

To help you focus on the proper feeling or quality of Tai Chi, we suggest that you keep in mind these three words:

Slow...Smooth...Soft.

Slow

The slow, gentle movements of Tai Chi help you to relax, release tension in your body and mind, and give you the time to focus on the proper feeling of Tai Chi. Moving slowly also provides enough time for you to pay attention to the various details of the individual moves.

Tai Chi is often called "moving meditation" because of the calmness, centering and mental awareness experienced during its performance. The focus of your attention on your movements, more readily done when you are moving slowly, causes you "to be in the moment", preventing your mind from wandering, a prerequisite for meditation.

The mental work necessary to perform Tai Chi indeed makes this an excellent mind/body exercise. It is well known that you can improve your mental faculties by challenging yourself with puzzles, card games, etc. The required details of Tai Chi also provide that mental exercise for you in a pleasant and easy manner.

Enjoy your practice sessions by taking your time with every movement. For most, it is a rare occasion when we allow ourselves to slow down and relax.

You will find your own innate rhythm which will feel appropriately slow for you. If your balance is challenged too vigorously, or your movements take on a choppy appearance, then you may be trying to move too slowly. Adjust your speed to suit your individual comfort level.

There are many other reasons for doing Tai Chi slowly and these will become evident to you as you continue your practice.

Smooth

Smooth, flowing movements stimulate deep breathing, balanced shifting and stepping, improved flexibility and coordination, circulation and the enhancement of energy flow (Chi) to improve and maintain your overall health.

Relaxed movements tend to be smooth movements. Keep in mind the goal of moving in a smooth manner and you will soon become much more relaxed, releasing years of accumulated tension.

Soft

Soft means not trying too hard, or using excessive strength, during any movement.

You should feel gentle reaching and turning during Tai Chi. Think about relaxing into each movement, rather than forcing yourself to move in any extreme manner. This is completely different from many other systems of exercise where you are typically encouraged to work "harder" and to push yourself more and more to achieve your health goals.

Think about a modern seatbelt in your car. It, by design, restricts your movement if you move suddenly and forcefully, thereby avoiding or decreasing injury. Your muscles and tendons behave in a similar manner. If you attempt to stretch very hard, forcefully and quickly, your tendons will act to tighten up to reduce the possibility of over-stretching and causing injury. In essence, you are fighting yourself by trying to stretch too hard.

By moving softly and slowly, you avoid the dangerous potential stress to your muscles, tendons and joints, yet your muscles will gradually release tension resulting in improvements in flexibility and circulation without injury.

Tai Chi is extremely safe, when performed slowly and softly with conscious attention to how you are doing the movements and how they feel.

After each Tai Chi session, rather than feeling tired and having strained your muscles, you will experience a sense of relaxed well-being, of having exercised your body and mind, and finishing refreshed.

Tai Chi has these different characteristics and approach because of its foundation in the Chinese Taoist philosophy, the understanding and method of being in harmony with nature. The Taoist philosophy is a living philosophy and is actually absorbed into your being by performing the exercises with conscious attention, rather than thinking about it in an abstract manner.

If you feel *any* strain in your knees, back or neck, or at any joint, please stop exercising and examine the pictures and descriptions closely; you should never experience any unusual stress placed on any of these spots. In fact, Tai Chi exercises have a strong reputation for being able to improve many conditions that affect these areas.

Great emphasis has been placed in this book on learning and practicing Tai Chi in a safe and comfortable way to ensure that your Tai Chi experience is an enjoyable and helpful one.

Regular daily practice of Tai Chi can:

> Improve balance and coordination,
> Lower blood pressure,
> Deepen breathing,
> Improve circulation and give a boost to your immune system,
> Decrease stress and anxiety,
> Increase muscle strength and bone density, and
> Improve flexibility and endurance.

All of this and more while doing a series of beautiful, slow, soft and flowing movements without straining!

Wu Chi Tai Chi is the unique Tai Chi Form created by the Tai Chi School of Westchester, est. 1978 that is taught in this book.

Unlike many other forms of Tai Chi, Wu Chi Tai Chi provides all of the above benefits in a brief and easy to learn series of exercises. You will find that doing Wu Chi Tai Chi is a relaxing and enjoyable experience that you will look forward to from your very first day.

For maximum benefit and enjoyment, we suggest that you begin your workout with a brief meditation (2-5 minutes), followed by several Chi Kung exercises, and then continue with your Wu Chi Tai Chi Form.

Your entire workout should only take 15-20 minutes, brief enough to do every day, if you so desire. You will find all of these exercises clearly described and illustrated in the following material.

You may find it very helpful to do your exercises at the beginning of your day, to loosen up, or at the end of your day to wind down. However, schedule your workout to finish at least one hour before bedtime. Otherwise, you may find that you are actually very relaxed, yet too alert to fall asleep easily! Choose whichever time is most appropriate for you and make it a regular habit.

Most importantly, have fun on your journey to outstanding health and well-being and walk the path of Tai Chi in health, peace, and balance.

How to use this book

To get the most out of your Tai Chi workout, we offer the following suggestions:

Select an appropriate time to practice free from distraction. It may be at any time during the day when you can avoid any interruptions for a few minutes.

Wear comfortable and loose clothing. Usually, shoes are worn during Tai Chi exercises, but that is your choice and you are welcome to practice in socks or barefoot, if that is more to your liking. Just be sure that you are not working on a slippery surface.

Some enjoy playing soft relaxing music during their workout to create a soothing atmosphere. Make your session as enjoyable as possible. If you have fun doing your Tai Chi workout then you will always look forward to it. Remember, Tai Chi is a "mind-body" exercise, so mental attitude plays a big part in providing outstanding benefits.

You are welcome to read all the introductory material before beginning the exercises to familiarize yourself with the structure of this workout.

However, it is not necessary to go through the entire workout every time. You may occasionally decide to choose specific exercises that you feel will help you at that time. For instance, if you are feeling particularly stressed, you may choose to do the

Tai Chi relaxation and meditation exercises for a few minutes to release tension.

Likewise, if you have a specific physical area that you would like to work on, say a tight shoulder, then you can simply go through the exercises that would help that area the most. Look through *Appendix B Benefits of the Individual Exercises* to decide which exercise you need to practice.

Most students will find it easier to go through a few exercises at a time, rather than trying to do the workout in its entirety immediately. As you become more familiar with the exercises and conditioned by your practice, you should add more exercises until you are performing the entire workout.

Ideally, you should perform some meditation/relaxation before beginning your exercises. Follow a brief period of meditation with Chi Kung exercises. These exercises will work on specific areas of your body.

Continue with the Wu Chi Tai Chi Form, the flowing sequence of exercises. If you wish, you may also conclude with a brief meditation, either sitting or standing.

All of these exercises provide great results performed either seated or standing. Choose the position that best suits you at this time and gradually add standing movements, when appropriate.

In fact, initially some of the turning exercises are best done seated so that it is easier to feel and control the isolation of your upper body to your lower body. This increases the benefit of the turning by working only the muscles of your waist and back.

Certainly, if balance is an issue at present, perform your exercises seated, or a combination of some seated and some standing, until you see improvement in your balance.

Indeed, seated exercises performed with the correct attention and focus will help improve your balance by working on your level of relaxation, coordination, alignment, strength and flexibility. Remember, your body is a whole, not just parts, so everything is supposed to work together in harmony and balance. Your balance is quite strongly influenced by these factors, which can all be improved even while sitting.

Each exercise has a specific breathing pattern. Using this pattern will give you the best results. However, it is important to avoid straining, so if the given breathing pattern is too challenging at this time, breathe naturally until you are able to use the suggested breathing pattern comfortably.

Use *Appendix C Breathing Pattern for the Wu Chi Tai Chi Form* as an easy reference to check your breathing technique when you are ready to synchronize your breathing to the movements.

You will find additional information in *Appendix A Tai Chi Meditation and Relaxation Exercises* to help you continue becoming more deeply relaxed and centered. Doing relaxation exercises before your Chi Kung and Tai Chi Form will increase your enjoyment and benefit tremendously.

If you have tried Tai Chi classes, you may have participated in sessions of 45 minutes, one hour or even longer. However, it is not necessary, nor desirable, for seniors to perform Tai Chi for that length of time. These longer sessions are frequently very tiring, both physically and mentally, and when overly fatigued you will see a reduction in benefits, especially in balance.

Practicing for a few minutes daily is preferable to doing a lengthy workout on any one day. The Tai Chi exercises provide you with long-term cumulative effects; so a little, consistently done, goes a long way in helping you improve your health dramatically.

If you perform most of the suggested workout, then going through one session a day is certainly sufficient. If you decide to isolate and do particular parts or sections of the workout, then you may also choose to spread it out throughout your day, as desired. The total for the day should still be around 15-20 minutes in order to show consistent development.

Think about your Tai Chi session as a time to get away from your daily stress and to center yourself. The mental focus and clarity provided by Tai Chi is a mental "vacation" you can enjoy any time.

Another way to enhance your practice is to invite someone to join you in a session and share your Tai Chi experience. Many Tai Chi groups have been created by friends practicing and growing together. It is often the case that what one student doesn't understand, another may be able to clarify, so the result is that everyone helps each other to improve and enjoy their Tai Chi workout.

The beauty of Tai Chi is that it is a wonderful self-healing system, whether practiced solo or in a group.

Follow the order of this book; first, meditation, second Chi Kung exercises, and then the Wu Chi Tai Chi Form.

The format of this book makes it easy for you to simply put the book down at any page illustrating an exercise and follow the instructions while seeing the photos that accompany the exercise.

Periodically, review the introductory material until you feel that you understand clearly the basic Tai Chi principles. You will find that as you continue to practice Tai Chi, your understanding of these principles takes on deeper meaning.

At the back of this book, you will find additional information about reaching us by phone, mail or email. We welcome your comments and questions.

Learn about joining our "Senior's Health Tips Line" where you will continue to receive valuable information to help you live a healthy life.

You will also read about how you are invited to take a **Free** (magic word!) Tai Chi lesson with Master Domingo Colon.

Remember; take it one-step at a time. Enjoy the process of learning Tai Chi and gradually improving your body and mind. You will be delighted with the "new" you, peaceful and calm, moving with grace and balance, and full of life and energy.

Senior's Tai Chi Workout   (15-20 minutes)

Sitting Meditation   (3-5 minutes)

Chi Kung Energy and Breathing Exercises
Sitting and/or Standing   (5-10 repetitions each)

1) Touch the sky with your palms
2) The archer draws the bow
3) The golden lion shakes its mane
4) Reaching across your body
5) The rhythmic heart
6) The rising and setting sun
7) The crane kicks out
8) The white crane spreads its wings
9) The golden rooster stands on one leg
10) Body tapping

Wu Chi Tai Chi Form
Sitting and/or Standing   (1-2 repetitions)

1) Step to side
2) Shake out the sheet
3) Wave your hands like clouds, right
4) Wave your hands like clouds, left
5) Roll the ball back
6) Squeeze the ball and stretch forward
7) Withdraw your arms and push
8) Cross your hands
9) Conclusion
10) Wu Chi standing meditation

Meditation

Tai Chi uses many different meditations to help you clear your mind, begin to release tension and stress, and to become more relaxed, lighter and more flexible. By performing a brief period of meditation prior to doing your other exercises, you will enhance all of the benefits of your Tai Chi workout.

Wu Chi Sitting Meditation

In a seated position, keep your back straight with shoulders relaxed and down, head up and look straight ahead. Move slightly to the front of your seat, so that your back is not resting against the chair. In this position you can more easily concentrate on strengthening your muscles to maintain your posture

Place both hands in front of you, waist level, palms down.

Curve your arms gently so that your fingers are pointing slightly towards each other. Feel the roundness of your arms continue into your back, as if you were lightly hugging someone.

Imagine that there is a string attached to the top of your head, reaching up to the ceiling helping to keep your head up and neck straight.
(Figs. 1 and 2)

Close your eyes.

Your back is straight…head up... shoulders loose... and down.

Breathe slowly and deeply. As you inhale, imagine you are drawing energy into your body with your breath…this energy flows down the front of your body to your *Tan Tien* (a *Chi* energy center about 1 ½ inches below your navel).

As you exhale, visualize this flow of energy moving under your torso…then up your spine…to the top of your head…and down your face to complete a circle.

Continue breathing slowly and deeply for 2-3 minutes, following this flow of energy with each breath.

If your shoulders become tired, simply let your elbows drop slightly.

When you finish this meditation, allow your hands to float down to rest lightly on your thighs. Pause for a moment, enjoying your new state of deeper relaxation, before you continue with the Chi Kung exercises.

Notes:

This seated position will help you to become more aware of your posture and develop the postural muscles of your back to help support your body. The straight, yet relaxed alignment of your body will allow you to breathe deeper with less effort. Your head held gently up reduces stress in your neck and shoulders and back.

The arm and hand position in this meditation improves the circulation in your arms, hands and fingers. This position will also release tension in your neck, shoulders and upper back. You can see that we place a great deal of attention on this area, since this is where most people carry their tension.

The curved position of your arms will also cause a gentle stretch across your upper back to help relax the muscles between your shoulder blades. As these muscles relax, you will notice that your breathing automatically becomes deeper, without any strain.

Most people will, even in this short period, experience several indications that they have become more deeply relaxed.

Some of the more common descriptions are:

> Shoulders dropping lower
> Muscles becoming looser and softer
> Arms, hands and fingers tingling
> Hands pulsing
> Hands becoming warmer
> The appearance of the palms changing-looking pinker as more blood flows into the hands and fingers

These are all good signs of deep relaxation and improved circulation.

This meditation is also known as "The Microcosmic Orbit Meditation", referring to the circular pathway of energy flow around your torso.

Meditation
(seated position)

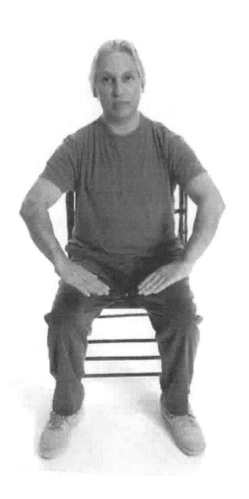

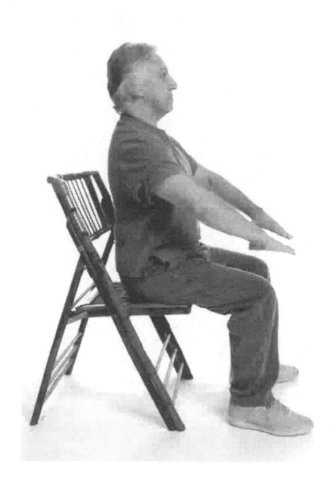

Fig. 1 Front view   **Fig. 2 Side view**

Chi Kung

These individual exercises work specific areas of your body and have well defined benefits. Chi Kung is frequently used as a warm-up before continuing with the flowing and connected movements called the Tai Chi Form.

The following beginning level Chi Kung set may be practiced individually or prior to your Wu Chi Tai Chi Form.

Chi Kung # 1   Touch the sky with your palms

Place both hands in your lap, palms face up.
(Fig. 3)

Inhale   Slowly, allow your hands to float up to chest level.
(Fig. 4)
Gradually, turn your palms out and then turn them to face overhead.
Stretch until you reach full extension, without straining and while still keeping your elbows slightly bent.
(Fig. 5)

Exhale   Relax your arms down and out to your sides.
(Fig. 6)
Return to the beginning position.

Repeat 5-10 times.

Notes   Your shoulders remain loose and down, even as you raise your hands. Feel a gentle stretch overhead and to your sides as you move your arms. Breathe slowly and deeply.

Chi Kung # 1 Touch the sky with your palms

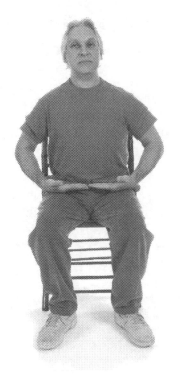

Fig. 3

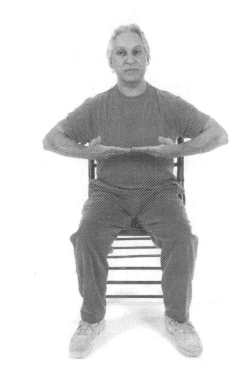

Fig. 4

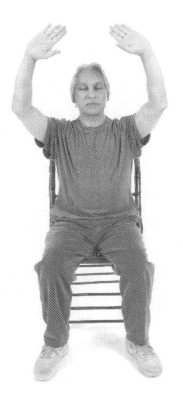

Fig. 5

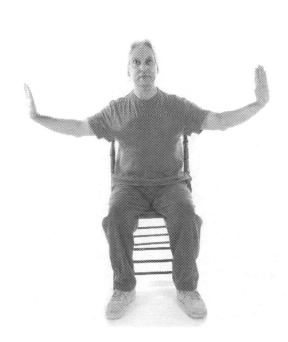

Fig. 6

Chi Kung # 2   The archer draws the bow

Place both hands in front of your chest, hands forming loose fists. Your hands are away from your body, gently stretching your upper back.

Inhale   Open one fist and stretch your arm out to your side, and push out with your palm, fingers point up, and thumb out to the side.

Your other hand also opens, but you push your elbow to the side, palm faces your chest, without straining and keeping both elbows slightly bent.

(Figs. 7 and 8)

Exhale   Bring both hands in front of your chest, closing them into fists once more.

Your back is again rounded and gently stretched.

Repeat 5-10 times to each side.

Notes   Keep your arms up throughout the exercise to work your shoulders.

Feel a gentle stretch at your wrists as you push your palm out, but do not force the movement.

Perform all exercises without straining. Your movement resembles drawing back on the string of a bow and arrow.

Chi Kung #2 The archer draws the bow

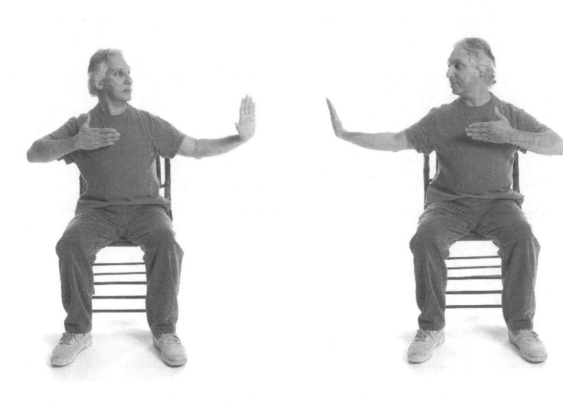

Fig. 7   Fig. 8

Chi Kung # 3 The golden lion shakes its mane

Place your palms lightly on your thighs.
(Fig. 9)

Exhale Lean forward until you feel a gentle stretch in your mid or low back.

While still leaning, turn your shoulders to one side.
Your head follows your shoulders.
(Fig. 10)

Inhale Turn your shoulders and head to face front.
Sit up, returning to the beginning position.
(Fig. 11)

Repeat 5-10 times to each side.
(Fig. 12)

Notes: Keep your back straight as you lean and turn.

Feel a gentle stretching of your spine the entire time, as if elongating your back. This is the feeling in Tai Chi called "suspension".

Do not push on your legs. Your hands rest lightly on your thighs to assist you in balancing and maintaining correct alignment only.

Turn only as far as you comfortably can without straining.

Chi Kung # 3 The golden lion shakes its mane

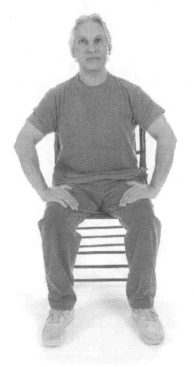

Fig. 9

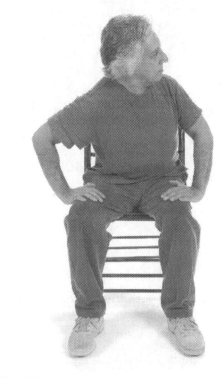

Fig. 10

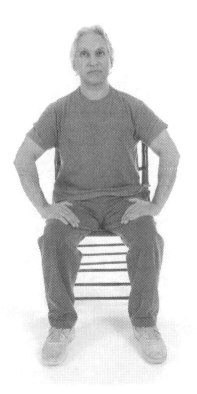

Fig. 11

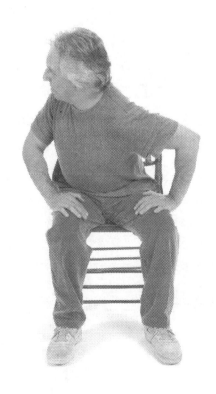

Fig. 12

Chi Kung # 4   Reaching across your body

Both hands rest at your hips, formed into loose fists. (Fig. 13)

Inhale   Raise one fist in front of your shoulder.
Turn your shoulders and reach across your body, as if punching to your side.
(Figs. 14 and 15)

Exhale   Return your fist to your hip.
Repeat with other fist.
(Figs. 13 and 16)

Repeat 5-10 times to each side.

Notes   Your shoulders stay relaxed and down while stretching.
Keep your elbow slightly bent and down to avoid locking out the joint.
Turn your torso as you reach across your body to feel a gentle stretch in your waist and back.
Your fists are gently closed; allow a little space in your hand, as if you are holding a pencil lightly in your fist. This hand position is known as the "hollow fist" to remind you to keep the hand relaxed.

Chi Kung # 4 Reaching across your body

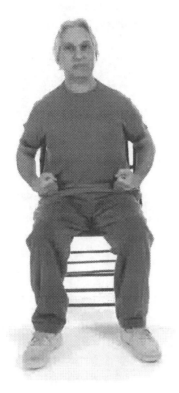

Fig. 13

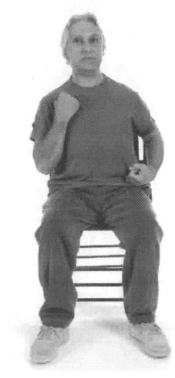

Fig. 14

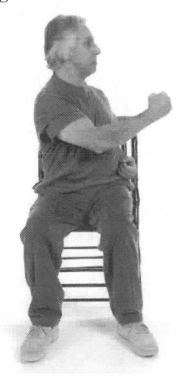

Fig. 15

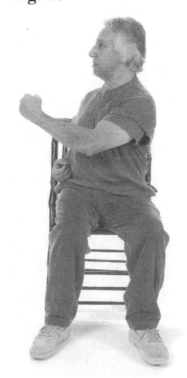

Fig. 16

Chi Kung # 5   The rhythmic heart

Touch your palms together lightly in front of your chest. (Fig. 17)

Inhale   Slowly, stretch your arms straight ahead until you feel a gentle stretch in your upper back and your chest muscles contract.
(Fig. 18)

Open your arms and reach back and down relaxing your chest.
(Fig. 19)

Exhale   Bring your palms together in front of your chest.
Form your hands into loose fists.
Draw your elbows back so that your fists rest at the sides of your chest.
(Figs. 18 and 20)

Repeat 5-10 times

Notes   Keep your shoulders down and relaxed throughout the movement.
Elbows remain slightly bent and down.
Breathe slowly and deeply without straining.
There is just a slight pressure between your hands when you bring your palms together.
Feel the stretch throughout your entire upper body, so that your back and chest are involved in the movement.

Chu Kung # 5 The rhythmic heart

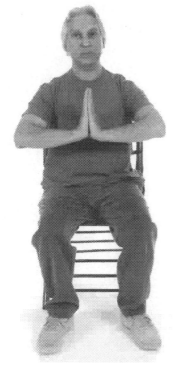

Fig. 17

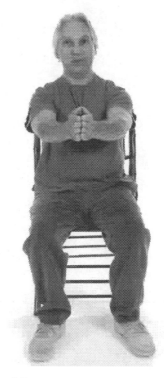

Fig. 18

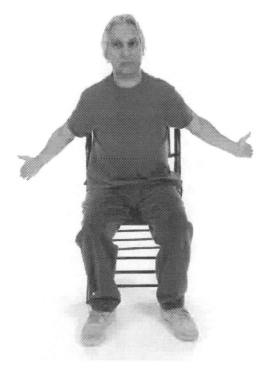

Fig. 19

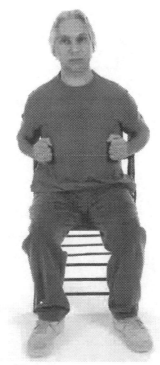

Fig. 20

Chi Kung # 6   The rising and setting sun

Place your hands in front of you and below your waist, hands gently curved, as if holding a large ball.
(Fig. 21)

Inhale   Slowly turn to one side, floating your arms up your side.
(Fig. 22)

Raise your arms overhead and look up towards your hands.
(Fig. 23)

Exhale   Relax your arms down to the opposite side, while turning your shoulders, and return to facing front.
(Fig. 24)

Repeat 5-10 times and then reverse the direction of your circles.

Notes   Your shoulders remain loose and down, even as you raise your arms.
Look towards your hands as you move so that your head follows the direction of your body and your neck stays relaxed.
Maintain a feeling of gently stretching, while keeping your elbows slightly bent, throughout the movement.

When you perform this exercise standing, keep your feet close together with legs straight, but not locked out. Allow your hips to turn to feel a gentle stretch throughout your entire body.

Chi Kung # 6 The rising and setting sun

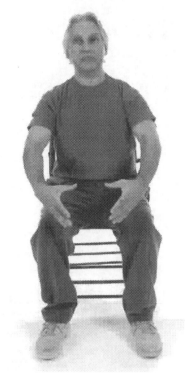

Fig. 21

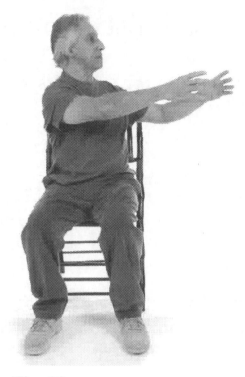

Fig. 22

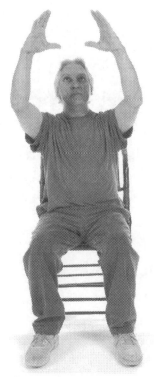

Fig. 23

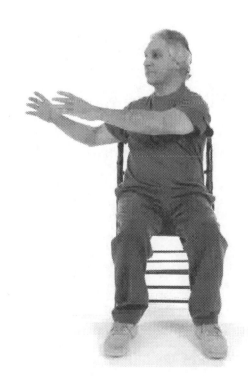

Fig. 24

Chi Kung # 7   The crane kicks out

Sit upright, your back slightly away from the back of your chair, feet flat on the floor.

Hold the armrests or sides of your chair to steady yourself.

(Fig. 25)

Inhale   Slowly extend one leg as if kicking forward.
Point your toes up, but keep your knee slightly bent.
(Fig. 26)

Exhale   Gradually and smoothly lower your foot to the floor and repeat with your other leg.

(Figs. 27 and 28)

Repeat 10 times with each leg.

Notes   Move smoothly and slowly to avoid undue stress to your knee or hip.

Point your toes up as you kick to feel a stronger contraction in your leg muscles.

The rest of your body remains relaxed. If you feel tension in your arms or shoulders, then you're trying too hard!

Chi Kung # 7 The crane kicks out

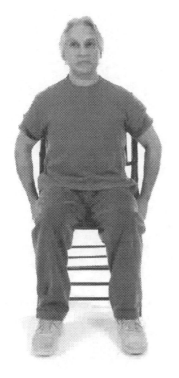

Fig. 25

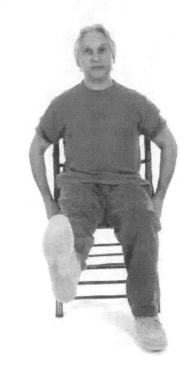

Fig. 26

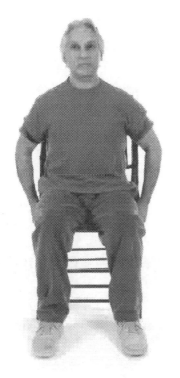

Fig. 27

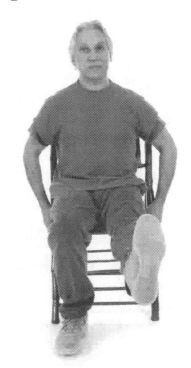

Fig. 28

Chi Kung # 8   White crane spreads its wings

In a standing position, hold the back or side of your chair to steady yourself.
(Fig. 28)

Step forward with the foot furthest away from the chair, while raising the same side hand to head level.
Now, step forward with your other foot to touch lightly with your toes.
(Fig. 29)

Return to start position slowly and repeat 10 times, and then switch to the opposite side.
(Figs. 30 and 31)

Note   Keep your knees slightly bent and in line with your toes.
Move smoothly and lightly, concentrating on good balance.
Your arm moves in time with your leg to help you improve your coordination.
Use the chair as support only to the degree that you need...avoid leaning on the chair if possible. You want to work not only on leg strength, but also on proper balance, so keep your body upright and relaxed.
Feel your weight solidly on one leg, with your heel heavier than your toes.

Chi Kung # 8 White crane spreads its wings

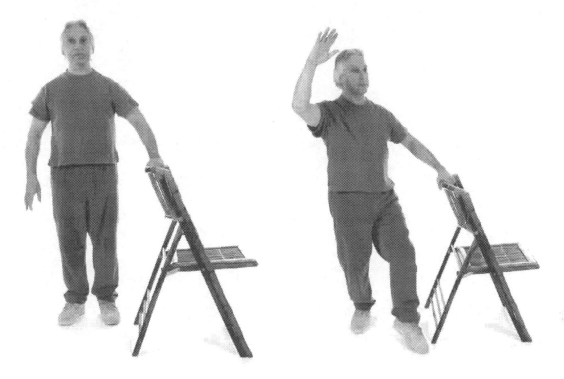

Fig. 28

Fig. 29

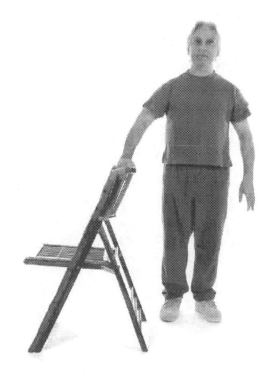

Fig. 30

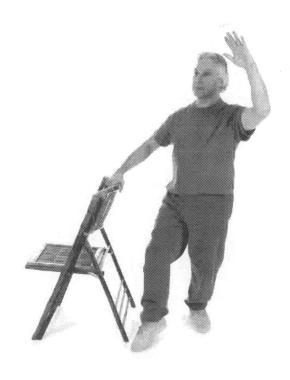

Fig. 31

Chi Kung # 9   Golden rooster stands on one leg

Continue holding your chair to steady yourself.
(Fig. 32)

Step forward with same side as hand holding the chair.
Pick up your opposite knee and arm, hand pointing up
and at face height, elbow down and relaxed.
(Fig.33)

Return to start position.
Repeat 10x, and then switch to the opposite side.
(Figs. 34 and 35)

Note   Step forward slowly, focusing on your feeling of balance,
stability and being grounded.
Keep your knee slightly bent and in line with your toes.
You do not need to raise your foot very far off the floor;
as soon as you pick up your foot, you are working on your balance.

Chi Kung # 9 Golden rooster stands on one leg

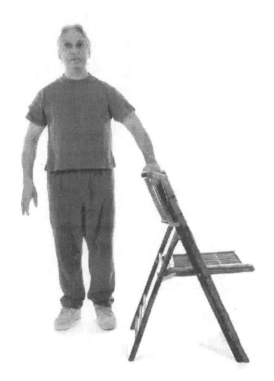

Fig. 32

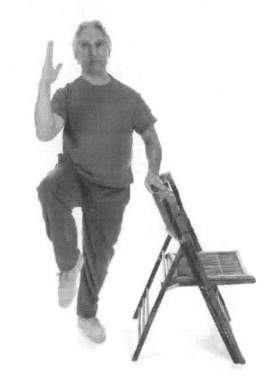

Fig. 33

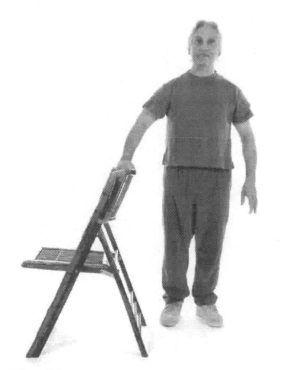

Fig. 34

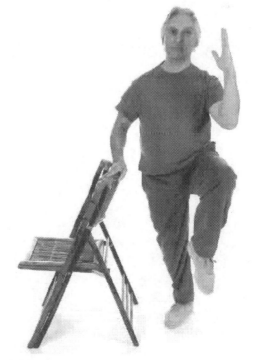

Fig. 35

Chi Kung # 10   Body tapping

Gently cup your hands. You are going to tap various areas of your body lightly to create a massaging effect that stimulates your circulation and relaxes your muscles.

Lightly tap on your arms, shoulders, waist, and around your torso, low back and legs.
(Figs. 36, 37, 38 and 39)

Repeat several times to each area.

Notes   Keep your hands relaxed and slightly cupped during the tapping.

Use enough force to feel the vibration within your muscles, but without causing any discomfort.

Tap carefully around joints.

Remember, this exercise is called "Body tapping", not "Body pounding!"

Chi Kung # 10 Body tapping

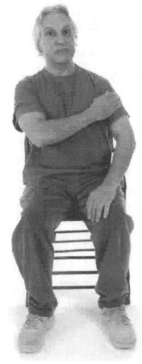

Fig. 36

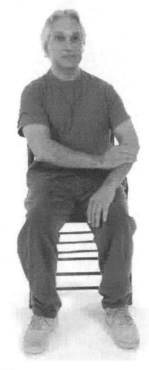

Fig. 37

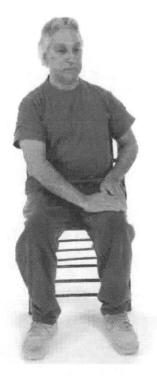

Fig. 38

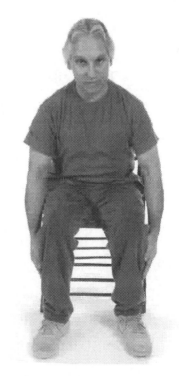

Fig. 39

Wu Chi Tai Chi Form

We suggest that you practice each exercise of this set individually a few times, until you feel more comfortable with the instructions and the movements. Then, when you feel that it is appropriate, add the next exercise.

There is no need to hurry to learn the series.

You can experience great benefits by practicing the individual moves; that is, one posture at a time, without the need to link them together or follow any particular order.

If you have an area of your body that you wish to focus on (i.e. very tight shoulders, waist flexibility and toning, leg strength, etc.), then it can be very helpful to concentrate on the exercises that you can feel working those areas.

If you would like more details about exactly which areas are worked by which exercises (or how those areas may benefit from a particular exercise), see *Appendix B "Benefits of Individual Exercises"* for an overview of the specific benefits for each Chi Kung and Tai Chi Form exercise.

There are additional benefits of performing the Wu Chi Tai Chi Form in its entirety; that is following the complete choreography. Since the benefits of the exercises are in fact cumulative and the sequence is designed to be progressive, after performing the entire Seniors Tai Chi Workout you will feel your breathing getting deeper and easier, your muscles relaxing and releasing tension and your mind become calmer and more focused.

So, keep in mind as a future goal to perform the entire Seniors Tai Chi Workout, with this book as your guide.

Feel free to experiment with how Tai Chi best works for you. There are many ways to do Tai Chi, and they are all correct as long as you keep in mind the basic principles of alignment, breathing, visualization and gentle relaxation of Tai Chi movements.

Although you are sure to feel some of Tai Chi's benefits immediately, other changes take more time and happen more gradually. In fact, very often you may not be the first to notice improvements. Instead, a friend or relative may comment on how you look "better, healthier", "move more gracefully and smoothly", etc. Then you'll reflect back to before you started Tai Chi and recognize the great strides you have made to living a more peaceful, healthy, and happy life

As Tai Chi becomes a part of your everyday life, the extent of your increased health and vitality will amaze you.

Wu Chi Tai Chi

Posture # 1   Step to side

Begin feet together, and arms relaxed at your   sides.
(Fig. 40)

Shift right, bending your knees slightly.

Lightly and slowly, step directly left into a shoulder width stance, feet parallel, facing forward, both knees bent and your weight evenly divided.
(Fig. 41)

NOTE

Your weight is evenly distributed between both feet, heels heavier than your toes. You should be able to wiggle your toes gently without losing your balance.

Feel the pressure in your mid-thigh area, not your knees.

Avoid twisting your knees; keep them in line with your toes.

Tuck your hips gently under you, as if sitting on a high stool or bench. This reduces the stress to your lower back.

Keep your back straight with your head suspended, as if a string from above were holding your head up for you.

Your shoulders are relaxed, loose and down.

Posture # 1 Step to side

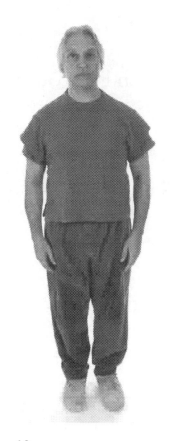

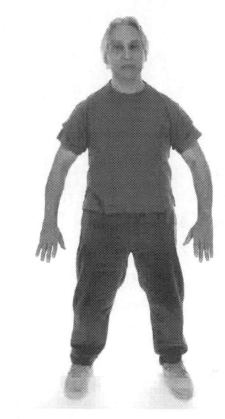

Fig. 40

Fig. 41

Posture # 2   Shake out the sheet

Raise both arms lightly in front to shoulder height. Your wrists and elbows are loose and down.
(Fig. 42)

Gently, stretch your arms forward, extending your fingers, but without locking out your arms.
(Fig. 43)

Draw your arms back toward your shoulders, with your hands moving parallel to the floor and elbows dropping down.
(Fig. 44)

Let your hands float vertically, fingers pointing up, as your arms come closer to your body.
(Fig. 45)

Slowly, lower your arms to your sides, fingers slightly up.
(Fig. 46)

Lower your hands to your sides, palms facing floor.
(Fig. 47)

NOTE   Shoulders remain loose and down. Keep elbows flexed, and feel a gentle stretch across your upper back as you reach forward.

This movement resembles shaking out a sheet, in slow motion, to make a bed.

Raise and lower your arms at the same steady slow pace. Feel as if you are moving softly in water.

Posture # 2 Shake out the sheet

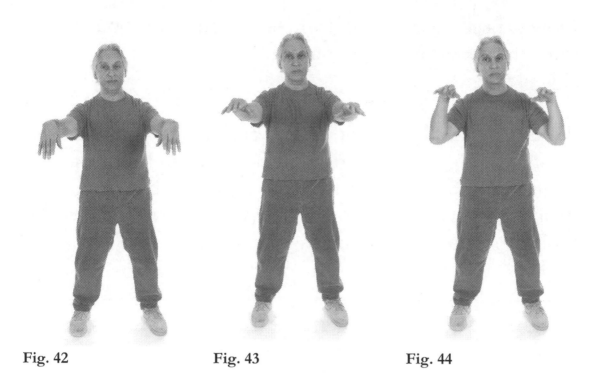

Fig. 42   Fig. 43   Fig. 44

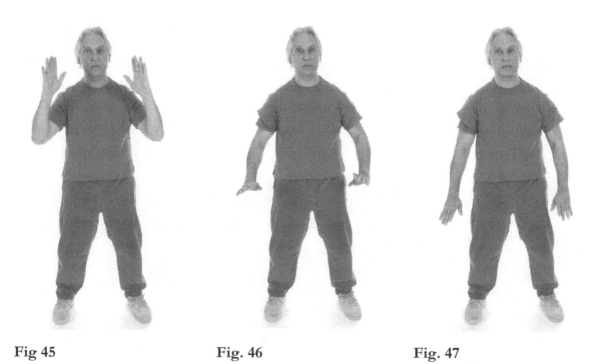

Fig 45   Fig. 46   Fig. 47

Posture # 3   Wave your hands like clouds, right

Slowly, raise your arms in front, as if you were about to perform "Shake out the sheet" once more.
(Fig. 48)

Turn your shoulders to your right side and continuing raising your right hand towards your right shoulder, palm facing down.
Your left hand also moves to your right side but at waist level, palm facing up. Curve your arms as if you are embracing a large ball with your arms and body.
(Fig. 49)

Imagine that you are rolling this ball over by lowering your right hand, moving it out and down and raising your left hand in and up until you have reversed their positions.
(Fig. 50)

Turn your shoulders to your left carrying the ball to your left side. Turn as far as you comfortably can, but keep your hips facing front.
(Figs. 51 and 52)

Note:

The name of this exercise comes from the visualization that each of your hands represents a soft fluffy cloud being gently rolled and moved across the sky by the wind.

Visualizations will help you become more relaxed and enjoy your Tai Chi practice more deeply.

Posture # 3 Wave your hands like clouds, right

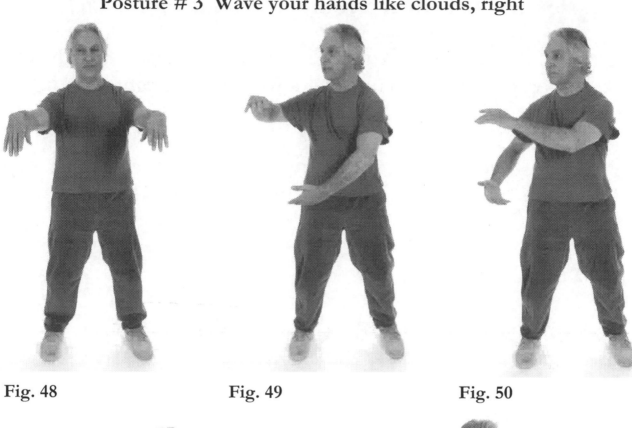

Fig. 48   Fig. 49   Fig. 50

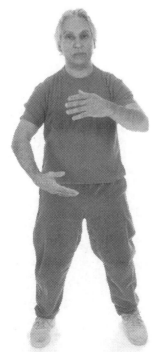

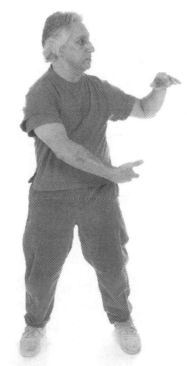

Fig. 51   Fig. 52

Posture # 4   Wave your hands like clouds, left

Roll the ball over at your left side, again reversing your hands, by moving your left hand out and down and your right hand in and up.

Turn your shoulders to your right side, returning the ball to the starting position at your right. Your hips remain facing front. (Figs. 53-56)

NOTE

Your hips remain facing front during the entire exercise.

Your weight remains equally balanced on both feet. There is no shifting during this exercise.

Round your arms, with shoulders relaxed and down throughout the movement.

Keep your arms soft. Move slowly and lightly. Remember, an imaginary ball has no weight!

Posture # 4 Wave your hands like clouds, left

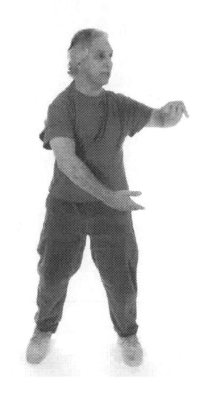

Fig. 53

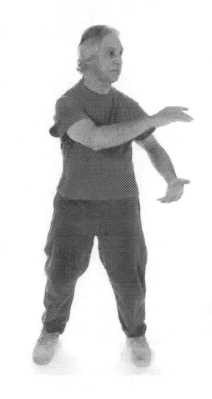

Fig. 54

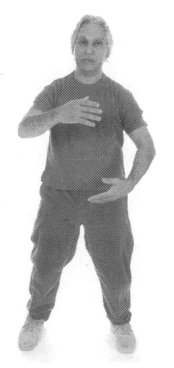

Fig. 55

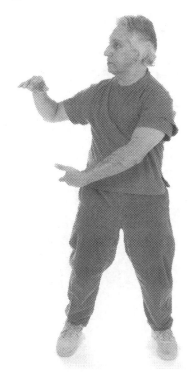

Fig 56

Posture # 5   Roll the ball back

Reach forward with both hands and shift onto your right leg.

Step back slowly and lightly with your left foot.
(Fig. 57)

Shift your weight back approximately 70% and turn your shoulders and waist left. Allow your hands to float down as if sinking in water and across your body until they are next to your left hip.
(Fig. 58)

NOTE

Your hands remain in the holding the ball position, but with your fingers now pointing down.

Step back as lightly as possible, like a cat, to concentrate on improving your balance.

Your arms and leg move at the same time to create a counter-balance for each other. This also helps you increase your coordination.

Your hips continue to face front.

Posture # 5 Roll the ball back

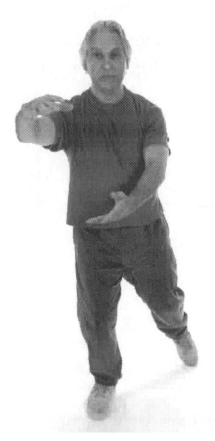

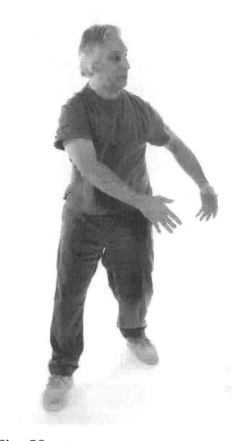

Fig. 57

Fig. 58

Posture # 6   Squeeze the ball and stretch forward

Slowly, let your hands float up to shoulder height at your left side, while maintaining the holding the ball position.
(Fig. 59)

Turn the fingers of your left hand up and allow your left hand to come forward so your palms are touching lightly, your hands are slightly cupped. Imagine that you are gently compressing the ball.

Shift your weight 70% forward. Turn your shoulders right and bring your arms in front of your chest stretching slightly forward.
(Fig. 60)

NOTE

Your shoulders remain loose and down as you raise your hands.

Your elbows are bent and pointing down throughout the movement.

Keep your knees in line with your toes and hips facing front.

Bend your arms slightly, as you shift and stretch forward. Feel a gentle stretch across your upper and mid back.

Posture # 6 Squeeze the ball and stretch forward

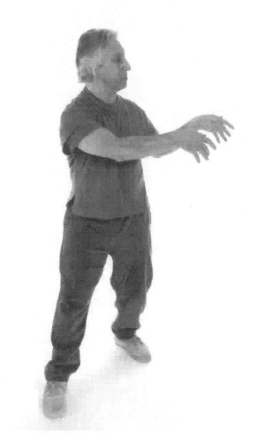

Fig. 59

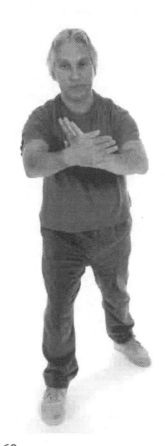

Fig. 60

Posture # 7   Withdraw your arms and push

Shift your weight 70% back onto your left leg. Your back comes into an upright and straight position, and you tuck your hips under you.

Open your arms wide, separating your hands, and with your hands coming more to your sides and back, at shoulder height.

Feel your chest opening as you move your arms.
(Fig. 61)

Lower your hands at your sides to waist level.
(Fig. 62)

Shift your weight 70% forward and push forward and upward with your palms at chest level. Your hands come closer together as you push forward.
(Fig. 63)

NOTE

Your shoulders are loose and down during this exercise.

Keep your arms slightly curved out and to your sides when you push forward to feel a gentle stretch in your upper back.

You want to feel your shoulders softly moving back and forth to improve shoulder flexibility and circulation.

Posture # 7 Withdraw your arms and push

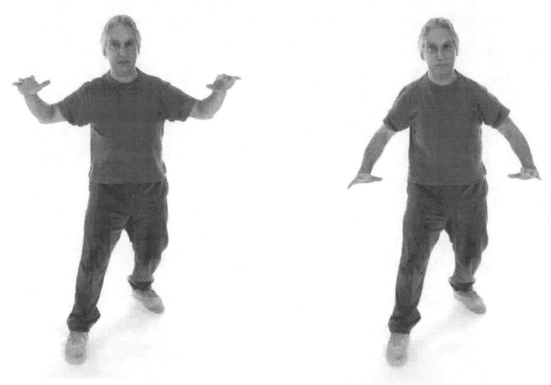

Fig. 61

Fig. 62

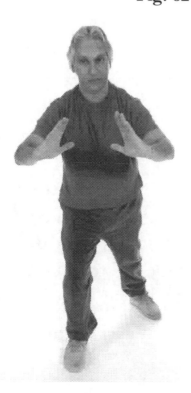

Fig. 63

Posture # 8   Cross your hands

Sit back onto your left foot. Raise your arms overhead and open your arms to your sides, palms facing front.
(Fig. 64)

Step back with your right foot into a shoulder width stance. Feel your weight sink back to balance on both feet, with your heels heavier than your toes.
(Fig. 65)

Lower your arms to your sides to waist height.
(Fig. 66)

Cross your wrists, left wrist in front. Palms face you.
(Fig. 67)

Gradually, raise your wrists to chest level, palms face down, then turn your palms to face you.
(Fig. 68)

NOTE

Raise your arms as you open them.
Your arms remain gently curved during the exercise.
Keep your arms away from your body when they cross in front of you to feel a gentle stretch across your upper back.
Your back is straight with your hips tucked under you and your head held up.

Posture # 8 Cross your hands

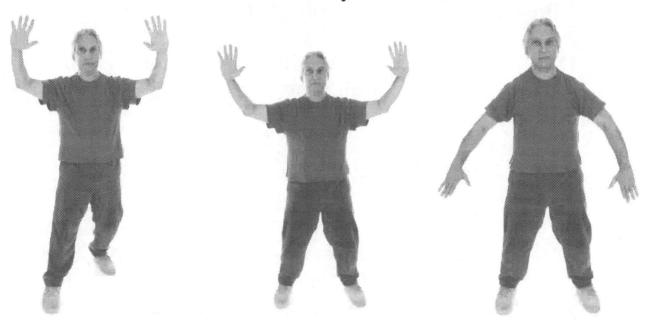

Fig. 64   Fig. 65   Fig. 66

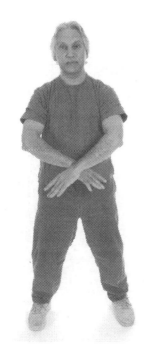

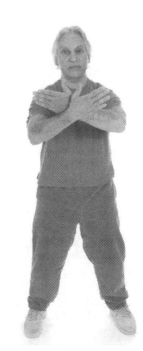

Fig. 67   Fig. 68

Posture # 9   Conclusion

Turn your wrists inwardly to lower your hands in front of your body as you gradually straighten your legs to stand upright.
(Fig. 69)

Lower your hands to waist level.
(Fig. 70)

Shift your weight onto your right leg. Step with your left foot next to your right, maintaining a parallel stance.
Slowly, lower your hands to your sides.
(Fig. 71)

NOTE

Your elbows remain loose and down.
Your elbows are slightly bent and pointing down.
At the end of the posture, your back is straight and upright with your hips tucked and your head held suspended.

Posture # 9 Conclusion

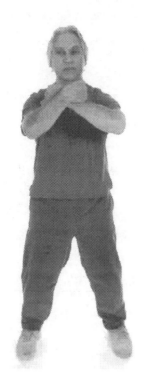

Fig. 69

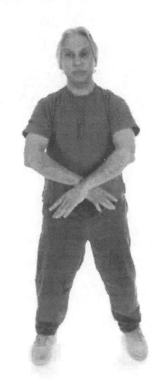

Fig. 70

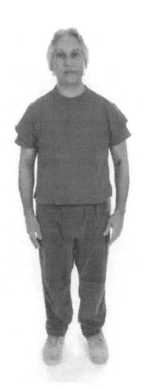

Fig. 71

Posture # 10   Wu Chi

Use this position to allow yourself to relax and feel the changes that you have made through your Tai Chi practice. Notice how you are breathing more deeply, yet with less effort. Feel the increase in circulation throughout your body, especially in your hands and fingers.

Appreciate how calm and stress free you have become.

Feel your body settle gently into your stance, with your heels heavier than your toes.

Hold your hands floating gently in front, as if held buoyant by water.

Suspend your head. Imagine a string holding you up at the center of your head.

Your upper body feels light and relaxed, while your lower body feels solid, rooted to the earth, like a tree projecting its roots deep into the ground.

Breathe slowly and deeply, feeling your Chi flowing strongly and smoothly through your body.

Hold this position as long as is comfortable for you and enjoy your new level of deep relaxation and peace of mind.
(Figs. 72 and 73)

Posture # 10 Wu Chi

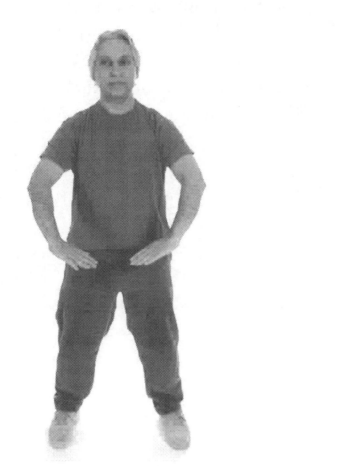

Fig. 72

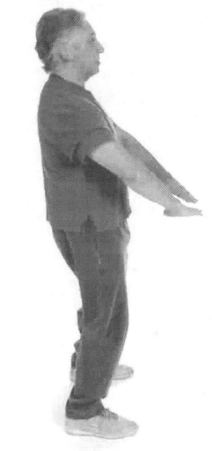

Fig. 73 (side view)

You have finished your Tai Chi Workout…coming full circle…returning to your starting position, and ready to experience your day with greater strength, balance and vitality.

Take the time to enjoy this new feeling of relaxation, calmness and energy that your Tai Chi has provided. The more you practice Tai Chi, the more you will feel all of these positive changes.

At this time, if you wish, you can repeat the Wu Chi Tai Chi Form by remaining on the same side or reversing the movements to perform a "mirror-image" form. (It is recommended that you practice on one side only until you feel more comfortable with the Form. Then, you may want to practice the opposite side as a variation. When you are able to perform the Wu Chi Tai Chi Form on both sides, your workout will consist of meditation, Chi Kung, and the Wu Chi Ta Chi Form, right and left sides.)

Every time you do Tai Chi, you will notice new and more fascinating levels being revealed. Enjoy your ongoing journey into increased health, peace and balance.

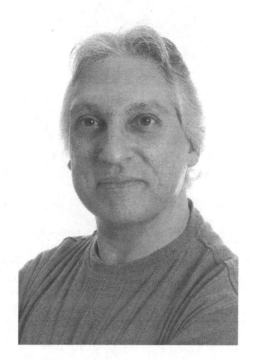

Master Domingo Colon

After investigating various exercise and health systems for over three years, Master Domingo Colon began his study of Tai Chi in 1965.

He found in Tai Chi a perfect combination of exercise, meditation, philosophy and self-defense, providing a superior balance of mind and body development.

One important requirement was that the system he chose to study would be one which he would be able to continue for the rest of his life, if he so desired, therefore the usual methods of conditioning were totally unsuitable...how many men get together to play football or basketball when they are in their 40's and 50's?

Tai Chi is an art that has been proven to be suitable for all ages, and the longer you practice the better you become!

He devoted over 18 years to studying intensely with three leading authorities of this art: Masters C. K. Chu, B. P. Chan and Wm. C.C. Chen, all teaching at the time in New York City.

By 1975, he had developed the necessary skills and was appointed Chief Instructor by Master C. K. Chu, while continuing to study and refine his understanding of Tai Chi's deeper aspects with Master Chu until 1983.

In 1978, he founded the Tai Chi School of Westchester, where he currently conducts classes in Tai Chi Forms, Chi Kung, Taoist Healing Techniques, Breathing Exercises, Meditation and Stress Reduction, Taoist Philosophy, Chi Development and Energy Channeling for Health, and Self Defense, Sparring and Weapons Techniques.

He has assisted many students in preparing to compete successfully in Tai Chi tournaments, and has served as a certified judge at these events since 1980.

Since 1971, Master Colon has taught numerous special courses for many Tri-State companies, civic groups, colleges, continuing education programs, hospitals and other health facilities. He has appeared many times on cable television and radio shows and is a contributor to specialized publications dealing with the martial arts and Chinese healing methods.

He has also designed specialized programs for seniors and individuals with special needs, such as Multiple Sclerosis, Parkinson's disease, Arthritis and many others.

Master Colon has an extensive and diverse teaching schedule, besides a full time schedule teaching at the Tai Chi School of Westchester in Bronxville New York, currently teaching at: St. Mary's Children's Rehabilitation Center, Hebrew Home for the Aged, Dobbs Ferry Seniors Center, Rye Brook Seniors Center, the Multiple Sclerosis Society, the Arthritis Foundation, Sarah Lawrence College, Stamford Hospital and Greenwich Hospital. Master Colon also assists and participates in scientific research to document the many benefits of Tai Chi.

Master Colon also studied physical therapy, working primarily in sports medicine, and in 1992 was certified as an Adaptive Fitness Instructor trained to teach aerobic, strength and flexibility exercises to the physically challenged.

This unique and extensive background in Tai Chi and physical therapy allows Master Colon to teach a highly effective and safe synthesis of Eastern and Western healing methods.

In 2003, Master Colon presented a comprehensive program for Tai Chi instructors, *"Teaching Tai Chi to Specialized Populations"* to assist Tai Chi teachers in effectively adapting Tai Chi for specific health conditions and circumstances.

Having taught senior's Tai Chi classes since 1980, Master Colon created special programs and teaching methods that are ideal for seniors, by carefully analyzing both seniors' needs and the fundamental principles of Tai Chi.

These programs take into consideration the special needs of seniors beginning Tai Chi, including possible limitations in range of motion due to arthritic conditions, discomfort from injuries, surgeries or illness, challenges to memory, and years of lack of exercise.

These programs are easy to learn, require only a modest investment in time, and provide many benefits. Seniors see a dramatic improvement in their balance, coordination, strength, flexibility, circulation, endurance, energy, mental focus and concentration after performing these Tai Chi exercises.

It is Master Colon's mission to help the many diverse populations with restrictions or special needs to experience Tai Chi's countless benefits easily, efficiently, and enjoyably.

Visit our website: **www.taichischool.com** for additional information about special events, articles, question and answer columns, exercises, philosophy, etc. updated frequently.

Your comments are welcome. We are happy to answer any questions and we personally respond to all email messages promptly.

Appendix A

Tai Chi Meditation and Relaxation Exercises

What is meditation?

Meditation may be briefly described as a self-controlled change in your level of consciousness with the purpose of increasing awareness, understanding, alertness, and psychological and physiological well-being.

During and after meditation, you will usually experience a deep feeling of relaxation of your body and mind. Your breathing will become deeper and slower, as your pulse rate decreases. The many other positive changes that occur are known as "The Relaxation Response".

Meditation is a state of body and mind that may be attained by various psychological as well as physiological techniques, which do not require a "mystical" or religious approach to achieve beneficial results. Whereas many religions employ various methods of meditation, Tai Chi does not restrict your personal beliefs in order to arrive at this higher level of thought and peace.

Properly practiced, meditation will not cause you to become "spacey' or out of touch with reality. Instead, you develop your concentration, focus and a harmony and balance of body and mind as you naturally progress toward an internal and external increase of awareness.

We are constantly exposed to stressful changes. Meditation is a useful tool to aid you in dealing with change, to avoid anxiety and the long-term accumulation of stress that often leads to psychological and physiological damage.

When we have any problem, it can usually be traced to a deep-seeded root cause of which we are not consciously aware. The present problem is just the "tip of the iceberg"; it is only the symptom of what is actually wrong. Meditation, although certainly not to be thought of as a panacea to solve all of your problems overnight, expands your awareness of yourself and others so that you may more clearly see and work with the true cause of your problem.

Meditation will be useful in preparation of your Tai Chi Workout by:

Calming you, allowing you to study and remember more easily

Begin the release of tension, thereby allowing you to move more comfortably and with improved balance and coordination

Moderating your emotions, not by repressing them, but by understanding the causes of your emotional reactions in daily activities, creating an enjoyable atmosphere for your workout

Meditation generates a more tolerant and easy going attitude that is not so easily disturbed by trivial external circumstances, so you will avoid feelings of frustration that often accompany beginning a new exercise program

Meditation will help you get in touch with "higher" levels of thought, providing you with a new way of perception that may give more meaning to your life.

Meditation is simple, relaxing and fun and helps create a positive environment for your Tai Chi practice so that you will look forward to doing your Tai Chi on a regular basis.

Preparation

Practice early in the day (ideally before breakfast), or at any time during the day (at least ½ hour after eating). Allow 5-15 minutes per session, but do try to practice on a regular basis. You gain best results by being consistent in your practice.

Wear loose comfortable clothing. If convenient, remove shoes, loosen belt, etc. to make yourself more comfortable.

Select an area away from people and free from distraction. Meditation is best practiced, at least for most beginners, alone and with a minimum of disturbance. Avoid drafty areas since you may find that you increase your body temperature during meditation due to the "relaxation response" and may even begin to perspire.

If appropriate, sit on a thick cushion or pillow in a full lotus position (right foot over left thigh and left foot over right thigh), or use any cross-legged position which is comfortable for you. You may also sit on a chair, separating your feet on the floor and placing your hands on your thighs, palms down. Sit slightly to the front of your chair so that you are not leaning against the back of the chair. Do not try to meditate while lying down; this is actually a more advanced position, since most beginners do not have the necessary control to remain focused and so simply become so relaxed they tend to fall asleep.

There are countless techniques of meditation, each giving slightly different results (i.e. there are special meditation techniques used by martial artists to generate exceptional strength and endurance).

The following are two basic beginning methods that anyone may use for improvement in centering, relaxation and stress reduction.

Progressive Relaxation

An overview of this technique is that beginning with your feet, you slowly tense and then relax each body part in turn. Become completely aware of each body part and any tension you may have in that area.

Then, slowly and gradually tense up only that body part. Maintain a mild tension for a few seconds and then allow it to relax completely. Proceed to the next body part and repeat this sequence until you have relaxed your entire body.

Follow this order, concentrating on each area for a minimum of ten seconds: Begin at your toes, then move up to your ankles, calves, upper legs, fingers, hands, forearms, upper arms, lower back, upper back, shoulders, neck, face and throat.

At the completion of this sequence, you may repeat this exercise or visualize relaxation as a wave of energy or warmth flowing from your feet up to your head. As you release excess tension, your mind will also gradually relax its hold on thoughts.

Breathe slowly and deeply and enjoy this new, deeper level of relaxation for a few minutes.

Counting your breath (1 to 6 count)

Simply focus on counting each inhalation and exhalation. (i.e. inhale and count 1, then exhale and count 2, continue to inhale...up to 6 and then begin once more be returning to 1)

Do not attempt to control your breathing; simply breathe normally. You will likely notice that as you become more relaxed your breathing will naturally become slower and deeper. Do not force that change...simply allow it to happen on its own.

Becoming more aware of your breathing focuses your mind and helps eliminate extraneous thoughts that interfere with meditation. If a thought comes to mind, just bring your attention back to your counting, starting at 1 if you happen to lose count.

Feel your body relaxing more and more as your mind centers on counting.

Either technique will help you to become much more relaxed and focused to function more efficiently in your life.

Appendix B

Benefits of Individual Exercises

Wu Chi Sitting/Standing Meditation

This meditation/relaxation exercise begins the process of relaxation, letting go of tension, and calming your mind. Meditation assists in the development of a stronger mind/body connection, creating a unique feeling of energy (Chi) flow through your body that you will experience in all of your Tai Chi exercises.

Your breathing deepens and you feel peaceful and calm.

The standing version will also release tension throughout your lower body. You will strengthen your legs and improve your balance, endurance and circulation.

Chi Kung Exercises

Touch the sky with your palms

Deepens breathing by relaxing various muscles in your torso and helping you expand your entire ribcage

Releases tension in your neck, shoulders and arms, and upper back

Gently works the muscles surrounding your shoulder joints to improve your range of motion in your shoulders. Increases circulation throughout your arms, hands and fingers.

The archer draws the bow

Stretches and relaxes your mid to upper back and shoulders

Improves breathing by coordinating the opening and closing of your chest to your breath

Strengthens upper back, shoulders, and chest muscles

Creates a gentle massaging effect stimulating circulation to the lymph glands located in the armpit area

Slowly opening and closing the hands increases circulation into the hands and fingers, while also increasing flexibility and hand and finger strength

The lion shakes its mane

Gently relaxes your waist and low back while working your shoulders and neck

Strengthens your low back muscles

Reduces pressure on the vertebrae in your back and neck

Improves posture and reduces fatigue

Creates a gentle massaging effect throughout your waist area, stimulating digestion and elimination

Also assists in improving breathing by releasing tension throughout your waist area, especially the abdominal, oblique and intercostals muscles around your ribcage

Reaching across your body

Increases flexibility in your waist, back and shoulders

Improves circulation throughout your torso and in your arms, hands and fingers

Strengthens the pectoral muscles of your chest, shoulder muscles, and upper back

Increases your arm, hand and finger strength

The rhythmic heart
Bilateral movements improves your coordination

Stretches your upper back and arms, while toning your chest muscles

Releases tension in your neck, upper and middle back

Improves range of motion of your shoulder

Strengthens your upper back muscles improving posture

Improves the circulation throughout your upper body, arms, hands and fingers

Breathing becomes deeper and more controlled when synchronized with the movements

The rising and setting sun
Loosens your shoulders, upper and lower back muscles

Improves the blood and energy circulation through your shoulders, arms and hands

Facilitates your lymphatic system circulation by massaging the lymph glands in your armpit, neck and torso

Improves your breathing by exercising your ribcage and associated muscles

The crane kicks out
Improves your balance

Strengthens your legs and hips

Increases your flexibility

Stimulates your lower body circulation

White crane spreads its wings
Strengthens your legs

Improves your balance

Improves your coordination

Releases tension in your upper body

Golden rooster stands on one leg
Improves the circulation of your lymphatic system by creating a gentle massaging effect to the lymph glands in your groin
Increases the strength of your hip flexor muscles
Improves the flexibility of your hip
Improves your coordination
Increases your balance

Body tapping
Relaxes the muscles of your upper body, shoulders, arms, hands and fingers
Stimulates the circulation throughout your upper body
Acts as a gentle "cool-down" for this series of exercises

Wu Chi Tai Chi Form

Step to side
This position is used to concentrate your mind, to focus your attention to direct your energy during the exercises.
Improves your balance and coordination
Strengthens your legs

Shake out the sheet
Gently relaxes your shoulders and upper back muscles
Releases stress and tension in shoulders and neck
Improves flexibility of shoulder joints
Improves movement of ribcage for deeper breathing

Wave your hands like clouds, right side

Releases tension in your shoulders and upper back

Strengthen and tones your waist and low back muscles

Improves your waist and shoulder flexibility

Improves your elbow and wrist flexibility

Acts as a gentle internal massage, stimulating digestion and elimination

Wave your hands like clouds, left side

Balances exercise to opposite side of your body

Releases tension in your shoulders and upper back

Strengthen and tones your waist and low back muscles

Improves your waist and shoulder flexibility

Improves your elbow and wrist flexibility

Acts as a gentle internal massage, stimulating digestion and elimination

Roll the ball back

Relaxing exercise for your shoulders

Improves circulation throughout your arms, hands, fingers, and lower body

Creates a gentle stretch of your upper, middle back and waist muscles

Massage to your internal organs

Improves your balance and coordination

Strengthens your thighs and legs

Squeeze the ball and stretch forward

Improves the strength of your legs

Improves your balance

Increases flexibility of your shoulder, arms and wrists

Tones muscles of your chest

Withdraw your arms and push

Strengthens ankles, knees, hips and pelvis

Improves flexibility of ankles, knees, hips and pelvis

Improves circulation in upper body, especially hands and fingers

Improves flexibility of shoulders and arms

Cross your hands

Increases flexibility of shoulders

Improves balance and coordination

Gentle flexibility exercise for elbows, wrists and hands

Gently stretches back and shoulder muscles

Strengthens chest muscles

Conclusion

Gentle exercise for your wrists, forearms and elbows

Continues the release of tension in shoulders

Increases circulation in arms, hands and fingers

Wu Chi

A relaxing position to end your Tai Chi workout

Acts as a way of centering yourself, strengthening your mind/body connection by letting you feel and absorb all of the changes that have occurred during your Tai Chi performance

Allows you to absorb this lesson into your being, making it an important part of your everyday life, necessary to allow all of your actions to be Tai Chi

Appendix C

Breathing Pattern of Wu Chi Tai Chi Form

Breathe in a smooth and relaxed manner. You should never feel any strain.

If the breathing pattern provided is too demanding at this time, you may either speed up your movements slightly to allow for more relaxed breathing, or breathe naturally (without following this breathing pattern) until you develop to the level where this breathing pattern is comfortable for you.

Breathe in and out slowly and deeply through your nose, if that is comfortable for you. Your tongue will naturally rest gently touching the roof of your mouth. This method allows your facial and throat muscles to become as relaxed as possible during the exercises, and facilitates the flow of Chi through the major meridians. This position can very often alleviate symptoms of temporo-mandibular joint syndrome (TMJ) pain.

This breathing pattern, synchronized with the movements, will enhance the exercise (by stimulating various circulations and working the deep layer muscles) and meditative benefits (by generating a profound level of relaxation and awareness) of the Tai Chi movements, so keep a goal of eventually following this method.

Begin with feet together... take a deep breath... inhale.

Exhale 1) Step to side

2) Shake out the sheet
Inhale a) Raise your arms and stretch forward
Exhale b) Draw your arms back
Inhale c) Raise your hands
Exhale d) Lower your hands

3) Wave hands like clouds, right
Inhale a) Hold the ball
Exhale b) Roll the ball and turn to center
Inhale c) Turn to face left

4) Wave hands like clouds, left
Exhale a) Roll the ball and turn to center
Inhale b) Turn to face right

Exhale 5) Roll the ball back

Inhale 6) Squeeze the ball and stretch forward

7) Withdraw your arms and push
Exhale a) Shift back and draw your arms back
Inhale b) Shift forward and push forward

8) Cross your hands
Exhale a) Stepping back and crossing your wrists
Inhale b) Raise your crossed wrists

Exhale 9) Conclusion-lower your hands, step feet together
10) Wu Chi-breathe slowly and deeply naturally

Glossary

Chi

Chi is the life energy that must circulate freely throughout our body and mind for optimum health and well-being;

Chi may also refer to breathing and the energy that is associated with the breath

Chi Kung

This is a type of Chinese exercise focusing on building, conserving and circulating Chi in your body for health and longevity. Tai Chi Forms are sometimes thought of as a series of Chi Kung exercises, one flowing into the next.

Meditation

The state of increased awareness and relaxation generated by specific techniques of visualization, breathing and/or movements; meditation can be used to enhance the psychological and physiological effects of Tai Chi.

Relaxation

Maintaining a position, or performing a movement, with a minimum of effort, while adhering to specific alignments, weight distribution, breathing technique, etc. for optimum health.

Suspension and Rooting or Sinking

The visualization of your head held as if suspended from above by a string (suspension) and the weight of your body sinking or dropping down into your legs and into the ground like a tree growing deeper roots (rooting or sinking)

This visualization acts to improve your alignment, strengthen your postural muscles, and gain better control of your center of gravity, improving balance. This practice is also necessary to improving your mind/body connection and stimulating the circulation of Chi in your body.

Tai Chi

Literally, "The Supreme Grand Ultimate", referring to the Taoist philosophy of existing in balance with nature

This is the source of the principles that form the basis of the Tai Chi exercises

The series of exercises, usually performed in a slow, soft and smooth flowing set also known as Tai Chi Chuan or Taijiquan

Tan Tien

A major Chi energy center located in the lower abdomen, approximately 1½ inches below the navel and a third of the way towards the spine

Used as a focus for concentration and meditation

Used as a physical point of balance in stances and movements

Yin and Yang

The theory that everything is composed of complementary forces that have an innate dynamic balance

As an example, in physical actions, yin usually represents the more relaxed phase, while yang represents the more toned phase

Tai Chi is a superior method of understanding and arriving at a balance of these qualities to improve or maintain your health

Wu Chi

The state of emptiness before the beginning

Before the separation of yin and yang

Used to identify the beginning or introductory level of our Tai Chi Forms.

Other Resources and how to reach us

Make learning Tai Chi as easy as possible, with our training videos.

Vol. 1   Fundamentals of Tai Chi
             Basic Movements, Standing and Sitting

This video is suitable for anyone, any age, new to Tai Chi and is available in English and Spanish versions.

Fully detailed instructions take you step-by step through the beginning stages of this flowing and gentle art.

Sitting and standing exercises guarantee you easy, safe, and fun practice of Tai Chi.

Two complete 15-minute workouts, one sitting and the other standing, are included for your convenience.

$30 check payable to: **DOMINGO COLON**

Order by sending your name, address and telephone number to:

Domingo Colon
27 Milburn Street
Bronxville, New York 10708

or call (914) 337-3339 for more information.

See our website: **www.taichischool.com**
for future releases of additional books, videos, etc.

Feel free to visit our school whenever you are in New York.

Join our Health Tips Line

To receive periodic updates, health tips, exercises, personal response to your email questions, announcements, chat line, and a 20% discount for future purchases of our new books, videos, etc., please register by filling out and sending in this page.

Only $20 annually payable by check, money order or on our website through Paypal will provide you with valuable information by email or regular mail to help you lead a more healthy and balanced life.

(Please print clearly)   Date_____

First name _____Last name_____
Street Address

_____

_____

City/Town _____State_____Zip code_____
Email_____

How did you learn about the School?
this book_____website_____Friend_____phonebook___

other _____

Benefits you would like to receive from Tai Chi_____

_____

Check enclosed or register by visiting our website: www.taichischool.com

**Mail to: Master Domingo Colon
                    27 Milburn Street , Bronxville
                    New York 10708**

Take a Free Class
with Master Domingo Colon*

Tai Chi… Beautiful, Relaxing and Easy to do

Relax deeply, move with complete confidence, grace and control.

Attain peace of mind and transform yourself into the healthy, balanced person you've always wanted to be!

Experience what it's like to study Tai Chi with a highly experienced teacher who can easily communicate this health system to you

*Bring a copy of this book to receive one free class.
Please call to make an appointment

(914) 337-3339

or email

sifu@taichischool.com

Tai Chi School of Westchester, est. 1978
27 Milburn Street
Bronxville, New York 10708

Keep up with our exciting new learning materials

Check our website often:

www.taichischool.com

or

telephone (914) 337-3339

or

write us at:

Tai Chi School of Westchester, est. 1978
Master Domingo Colon
27 Milburn Street
Bronxville, New York 10708

Printed in the United States
By Bookmasters